Stan the Plant-Eater

By: Stephen Bedwell Jr.

Illustrated by: Syeda Jabeen Qadri

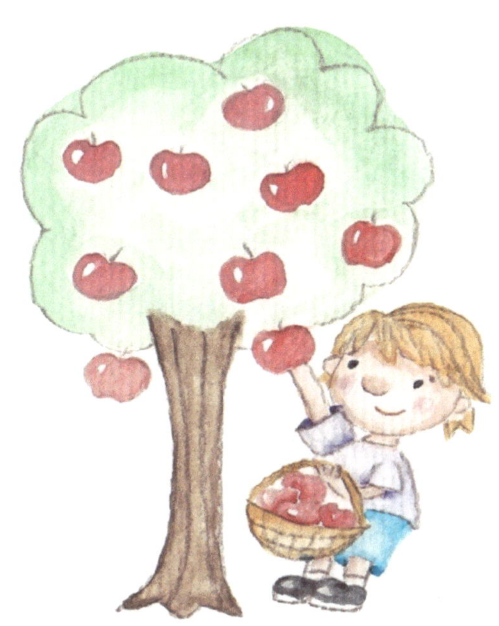

Dedicated to
a healthy and loving future
for all children.

ISBN-10: 1974262227
ISBN-13: 978-1974262229

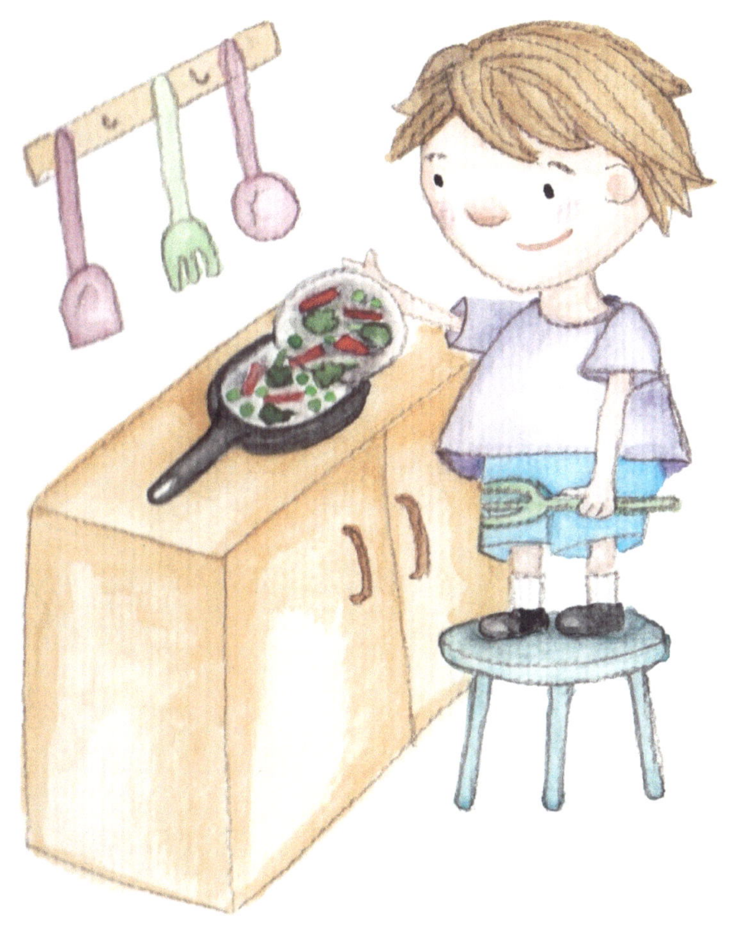

Who is that standing tall on a stool? It is Stan!

He's putting fresh plant foods into the cooking pan.

Stan really loves to eat.

Plant foods are always his favorite treat.

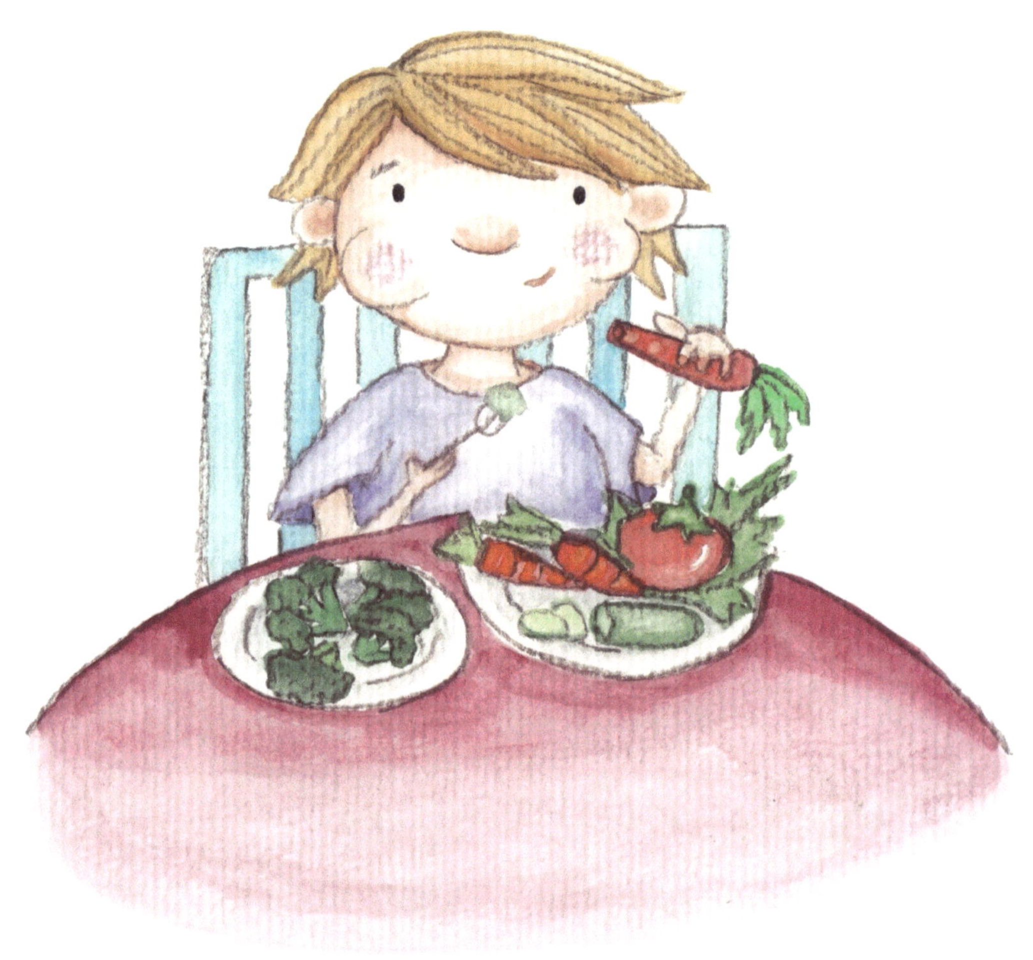

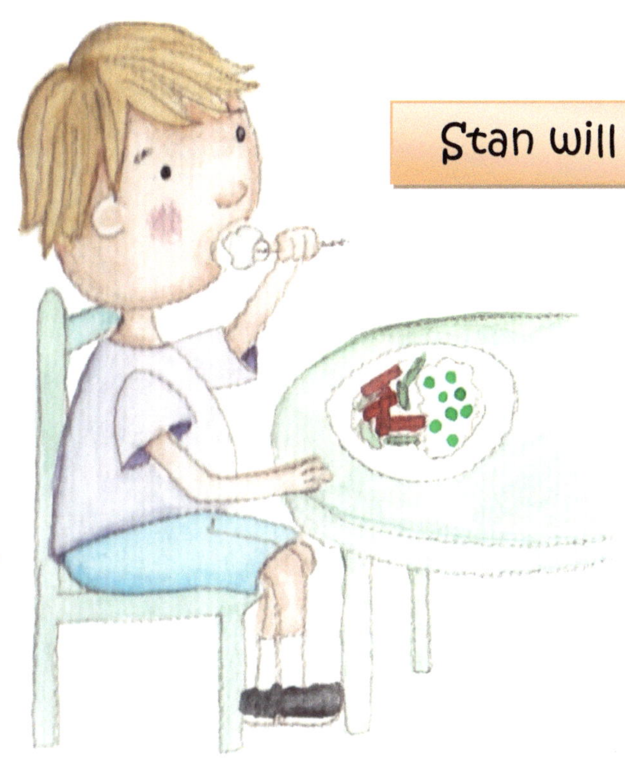

Stan will eat plant foods in a seat.

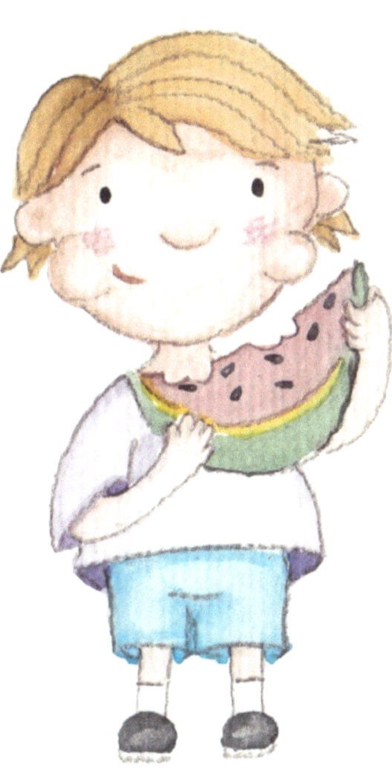

Stan will eat plant foods on
his two feet.

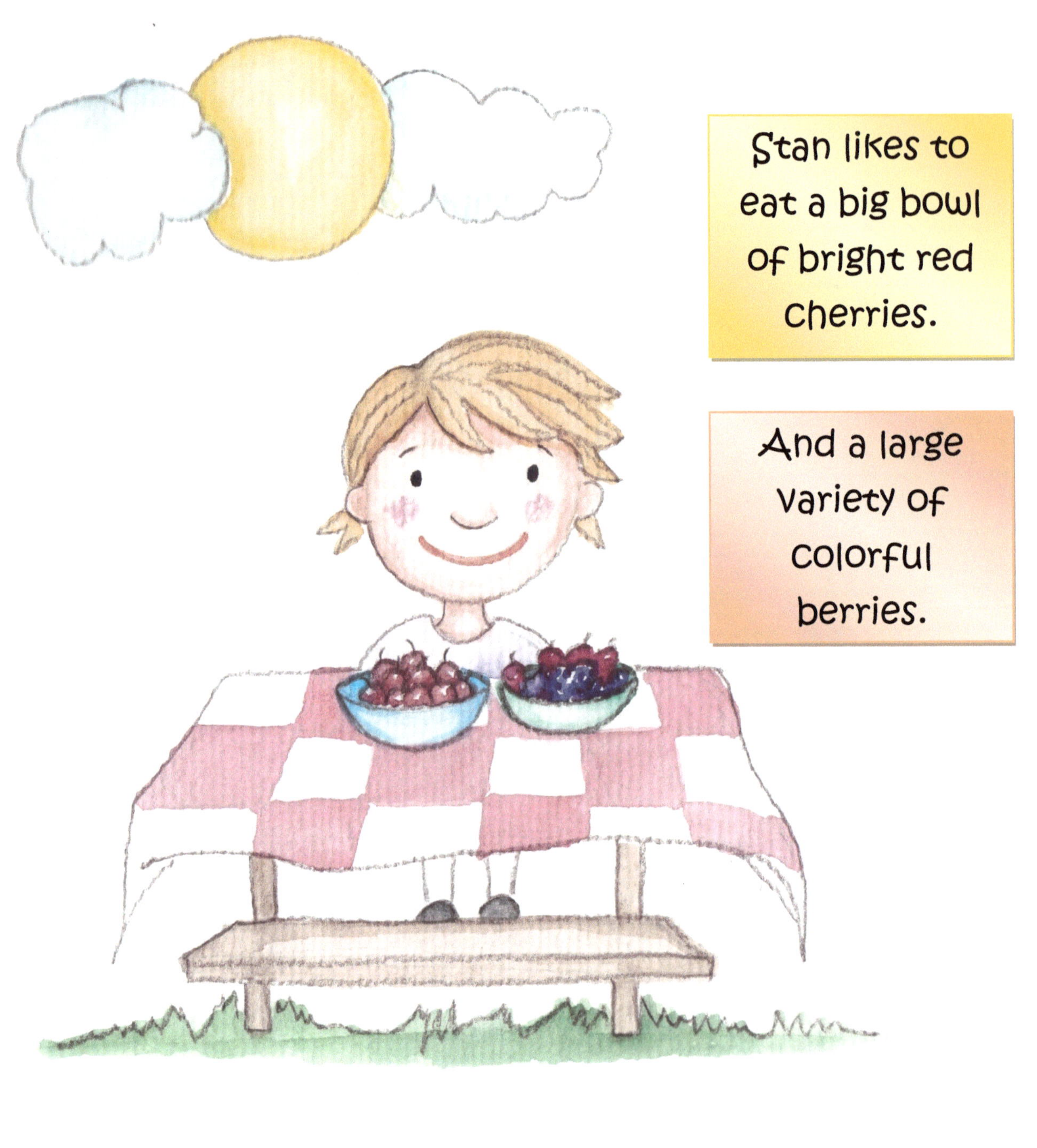

Stan likes to eat a big bowl of bright red cherries.

And a large variety of colorful berries.

Stan will eat some spaghetti noodles and tomatoes.

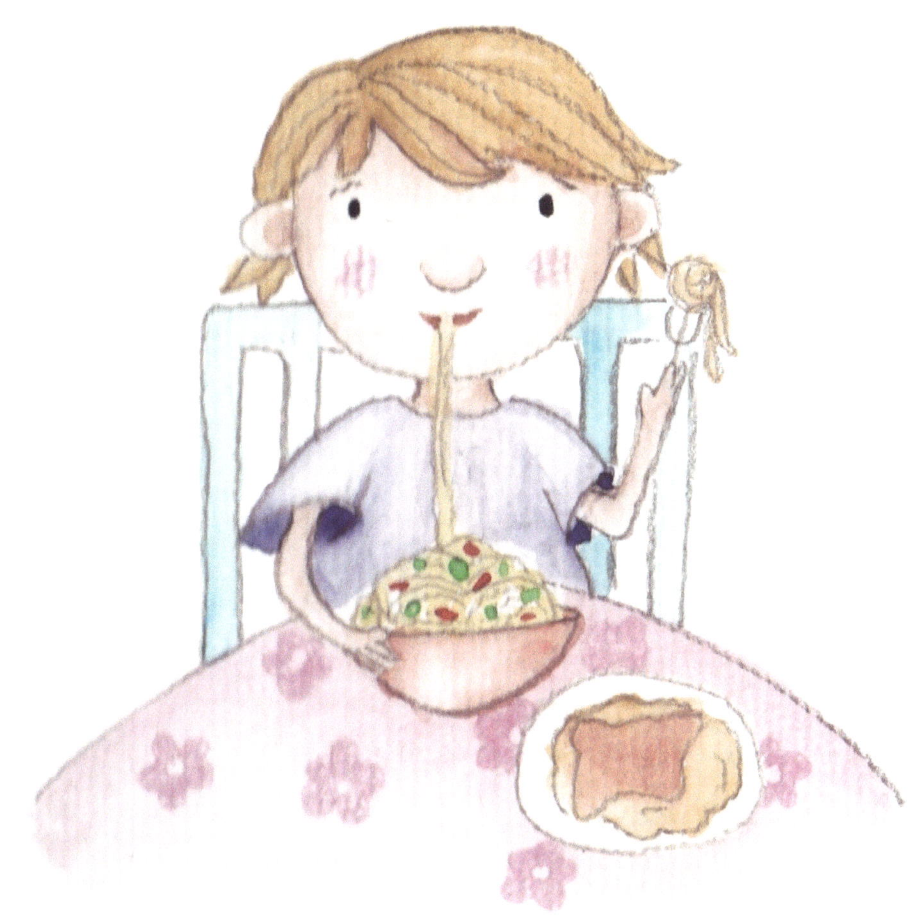

Or a giant helping of yummy mashed potatoes.

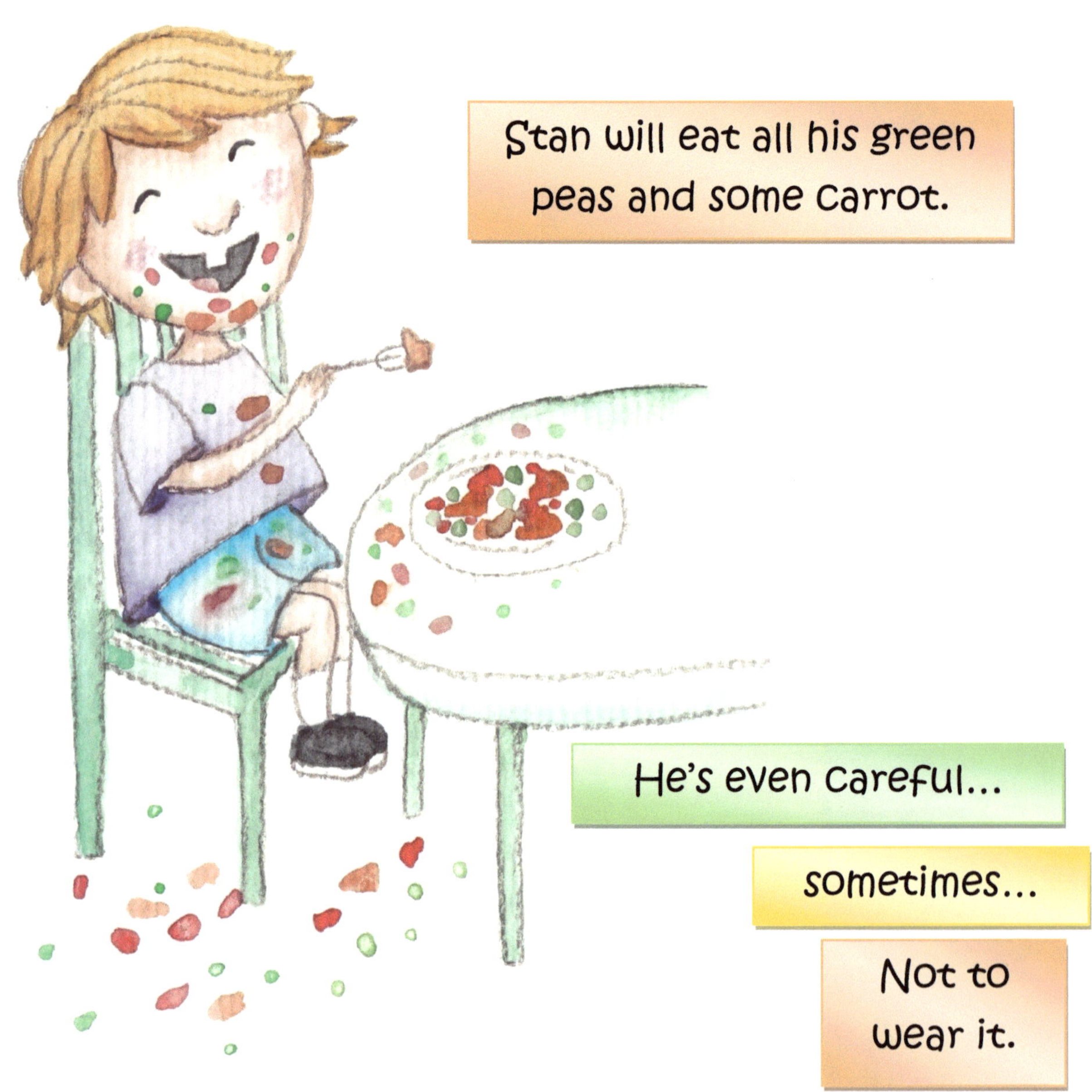

Stan will eat all his green peas and some carrot.
He's even careful...
sometimes...
Not to wear it.

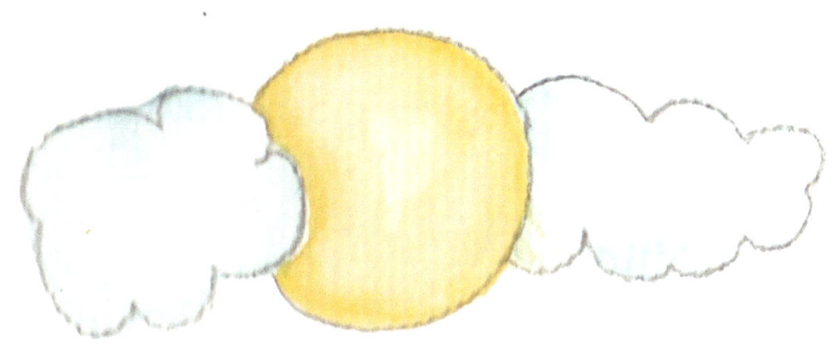

Stan really likes a breakfast of warm oatmeal.

He enjoys how full it makes him feel.

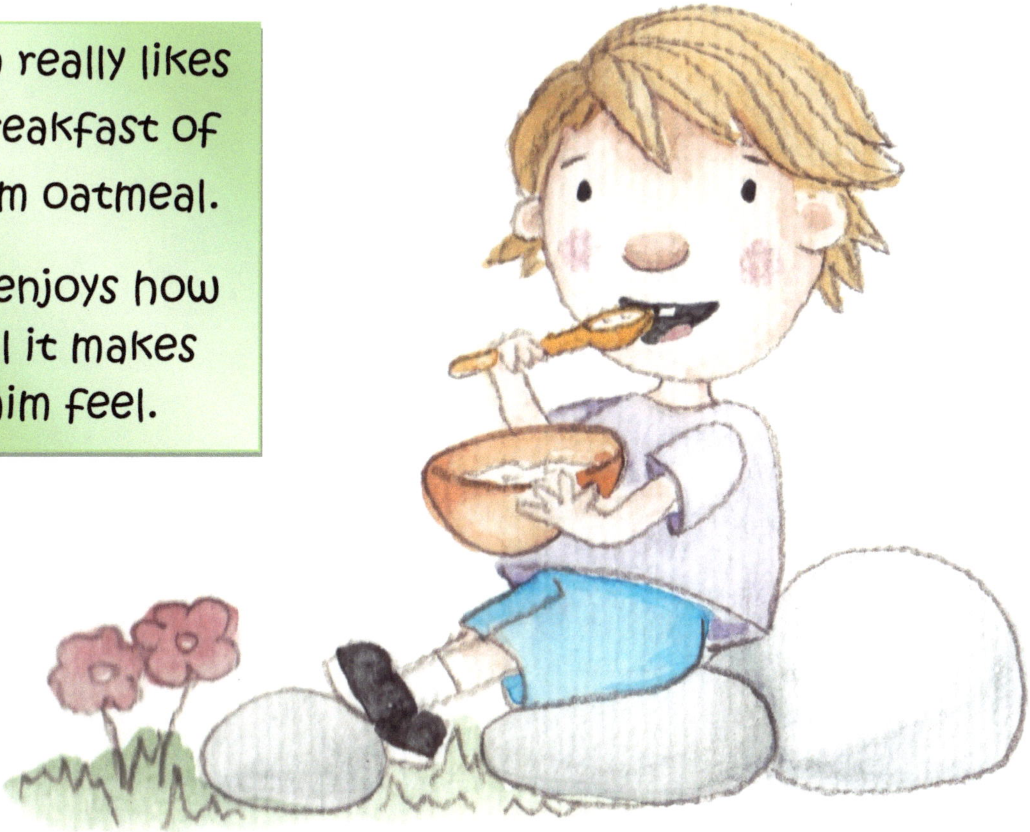

Black bean tacos are his favorite lunch.

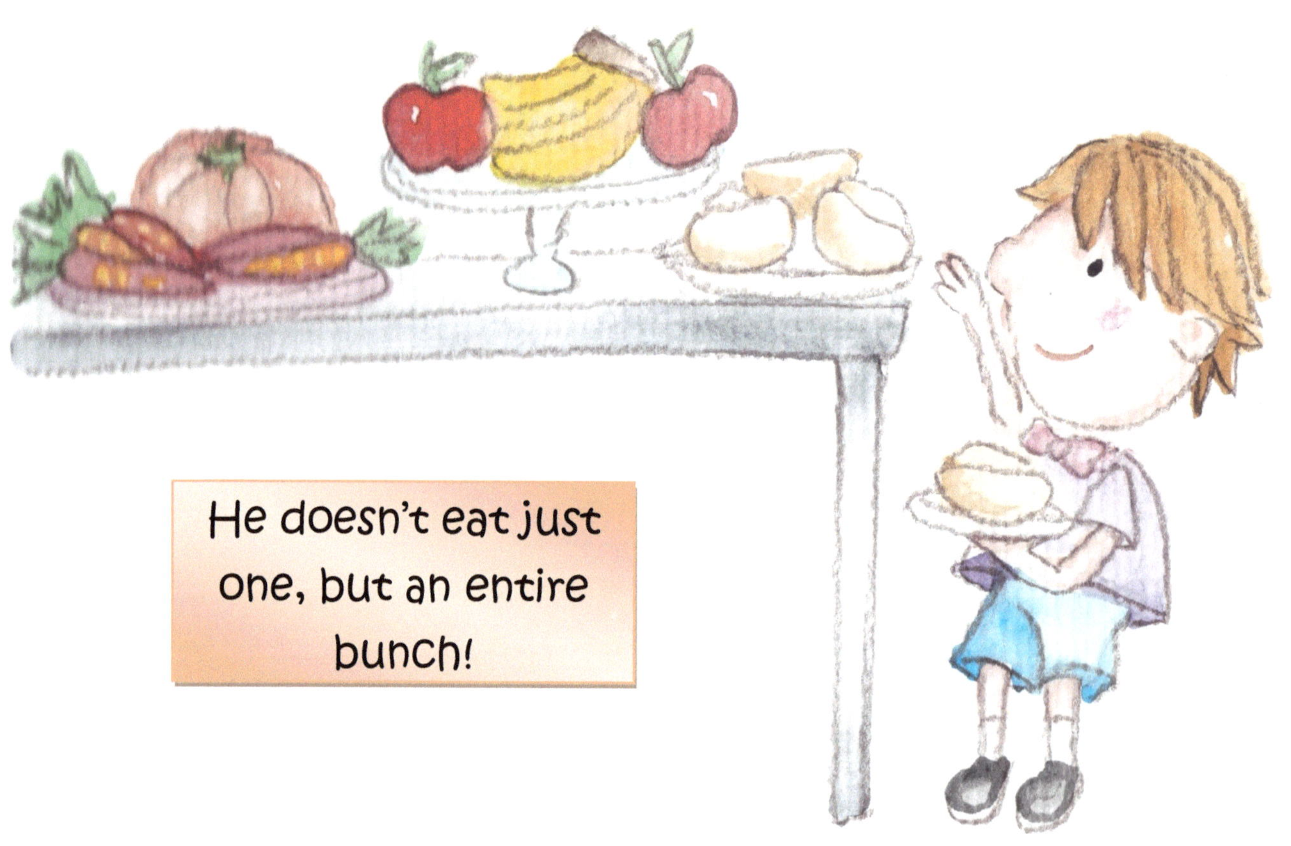

He doesn't eat just one, but an entire bunch!

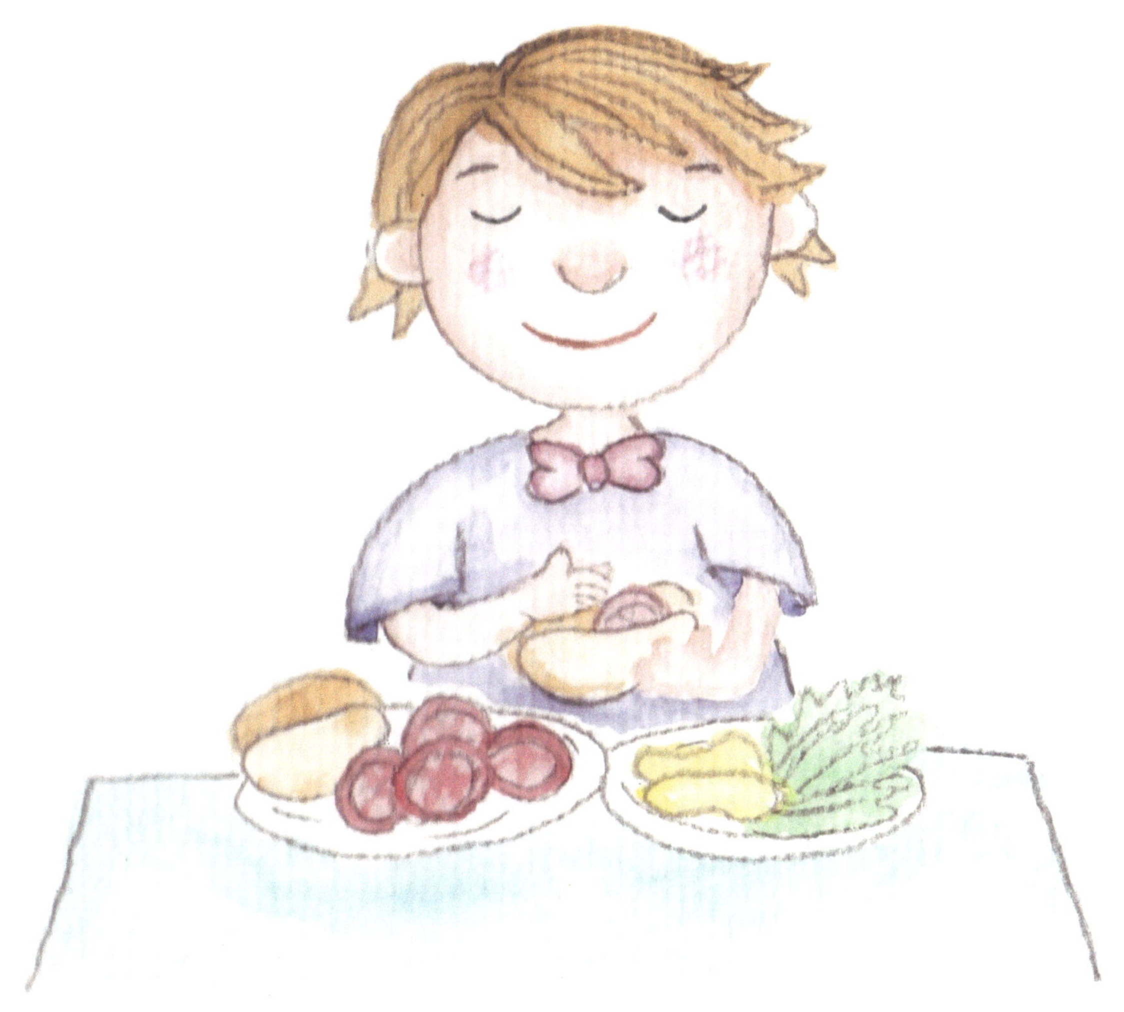

Stan will stuff his tacos with brown rice, crunchy lettuce, and tomatoes.

Sometimes he will even stuff in tasty, orange sweet potatoes.

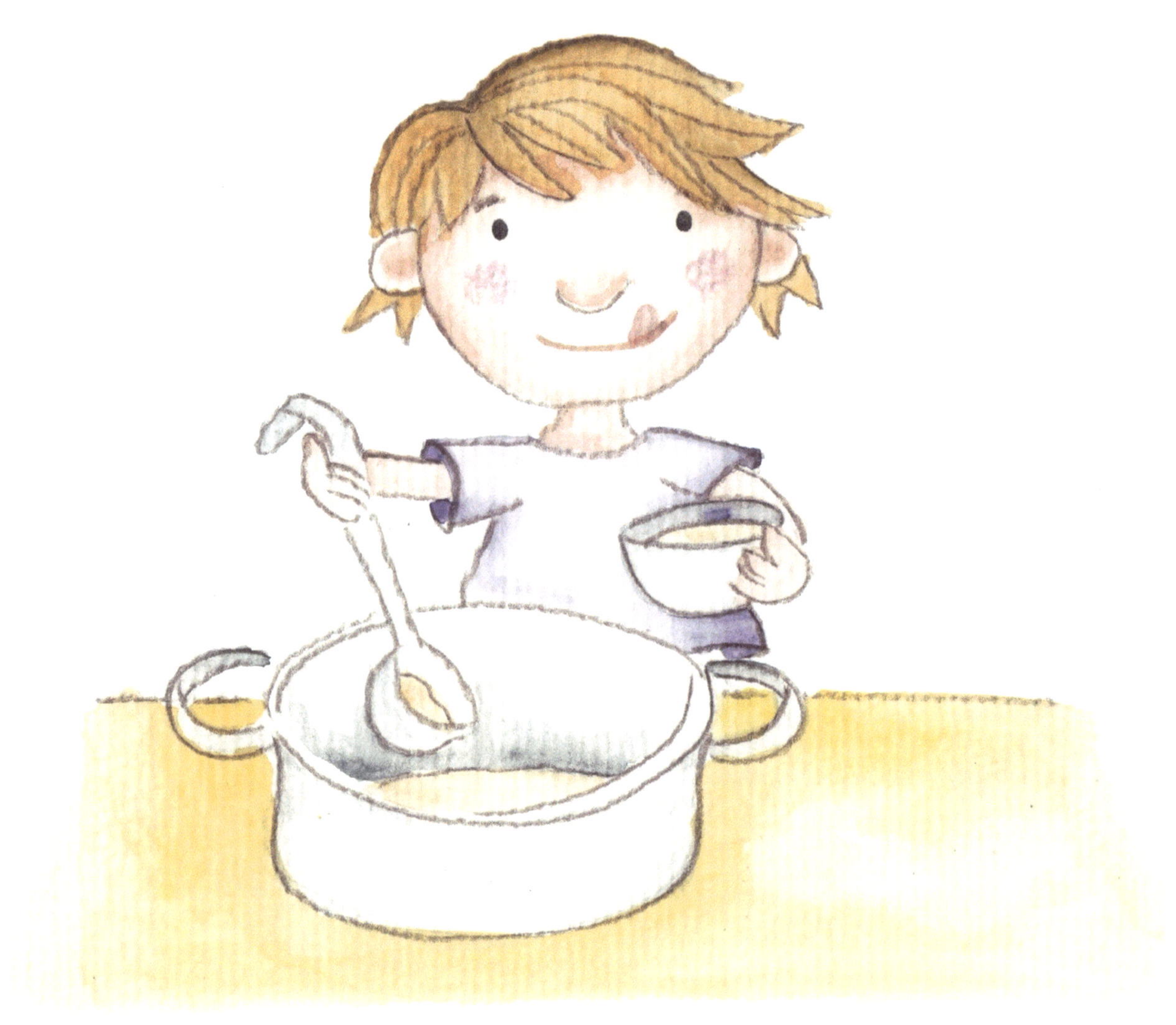

Stan's favorite for dinner is veggie soup. It's always nice and hot.

It is filled with many plant foods so Stan is sure to eat a lot!

Sometimes, he will almost eat what is in the entire pot!

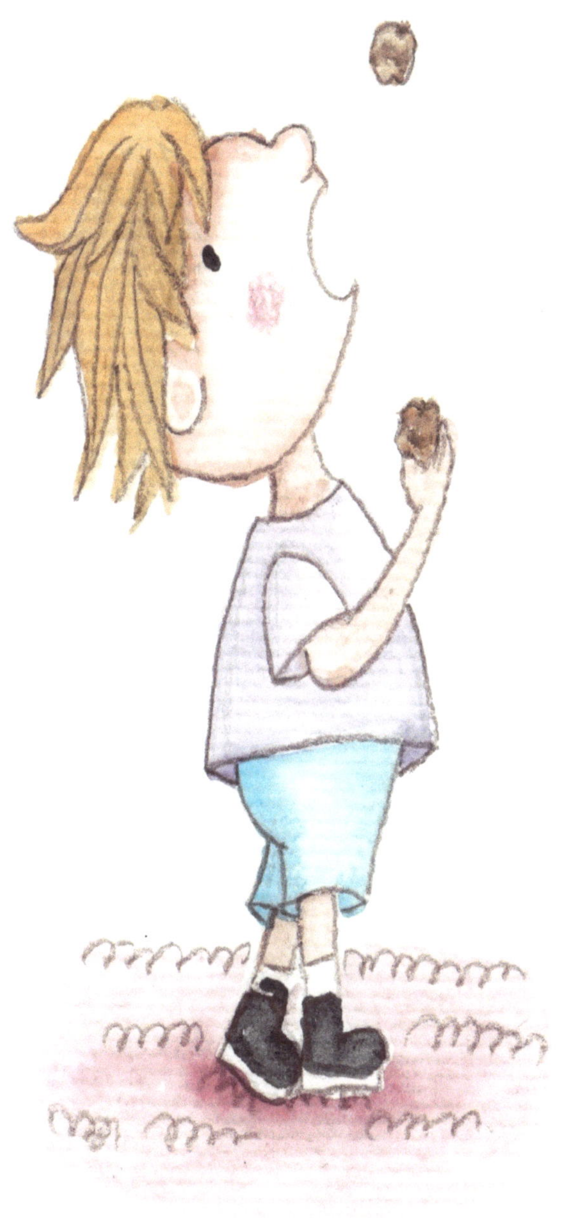

Stan loves to make and eat dessert.

He tries not to have it land on his shirt.

Stan takes raisins, nuts, and dates and rolls them into one big ball.

He finds eating this to be so much fun that he eats them all.

Eating all these plant foods makes Stan big and strong.

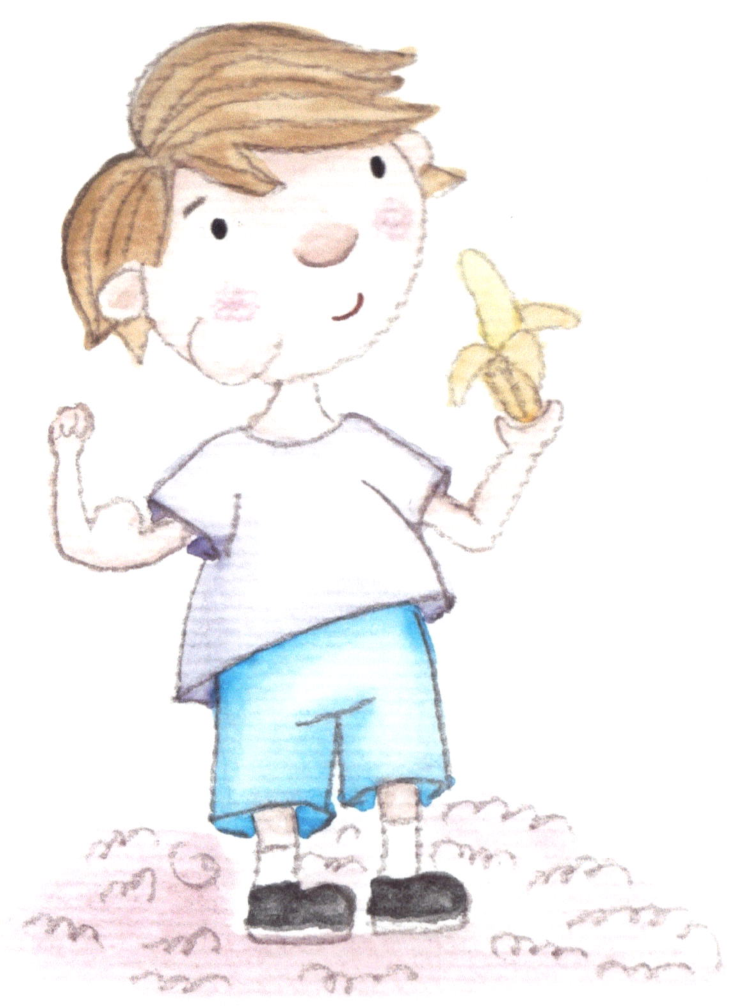

He could sit or stand and eat them all day long.

There are some things that Stan will just not eat.

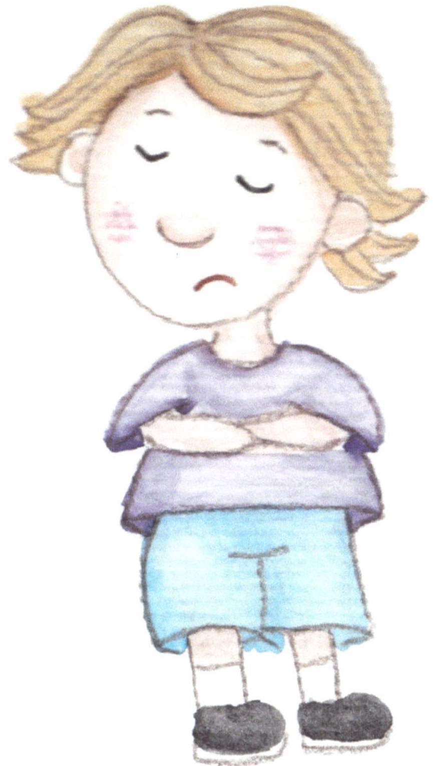

He will not eat these in a seat.

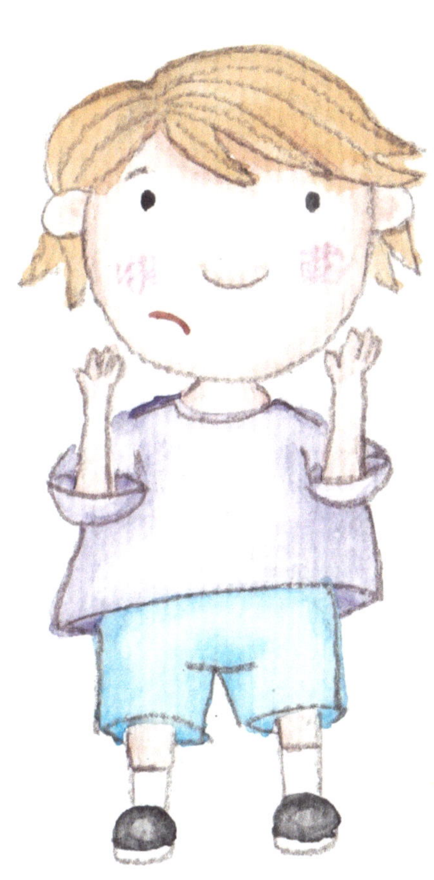

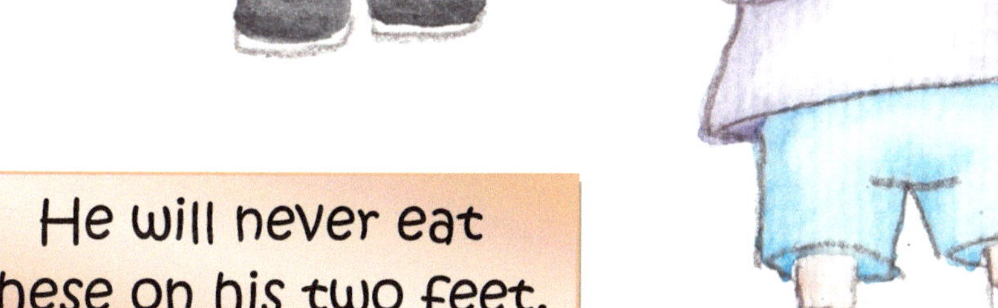

He will never eat
these on his two feet.

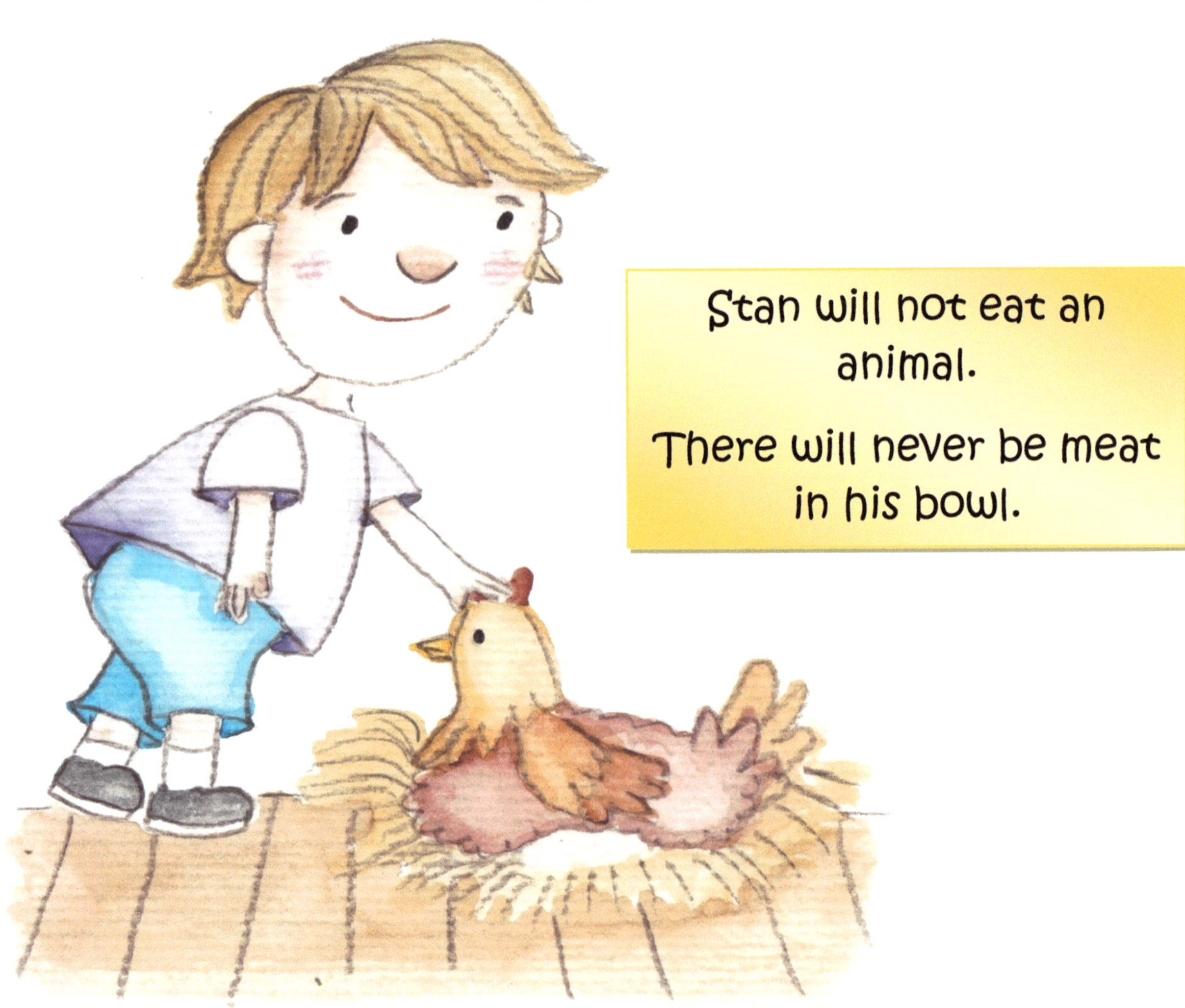

Stan will not eat a piece of meat.

He will never knock a chicken off her seat.

Stan will not eat an animal.

There will never be meat in his bowl.

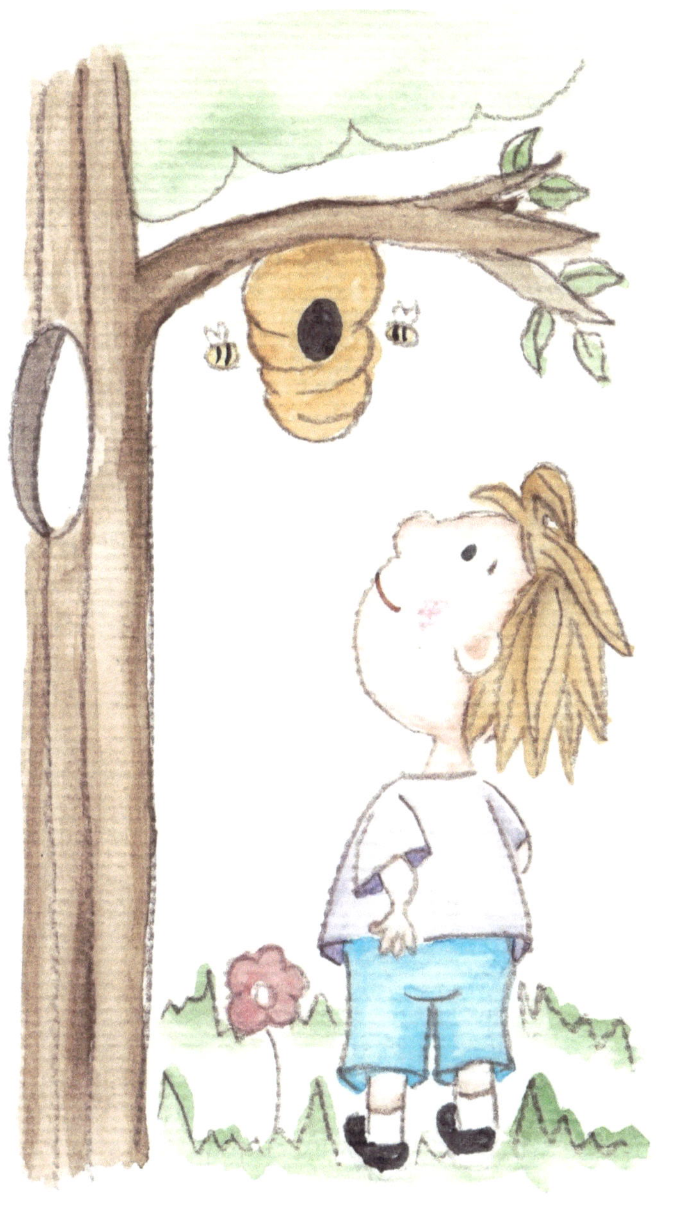

Stan will not eat a piece of cheese.

Nor will he steal from any bees.

Stan allows the bees to keep all their sweet honey.

He finds watching buzzing bees to be very funny.

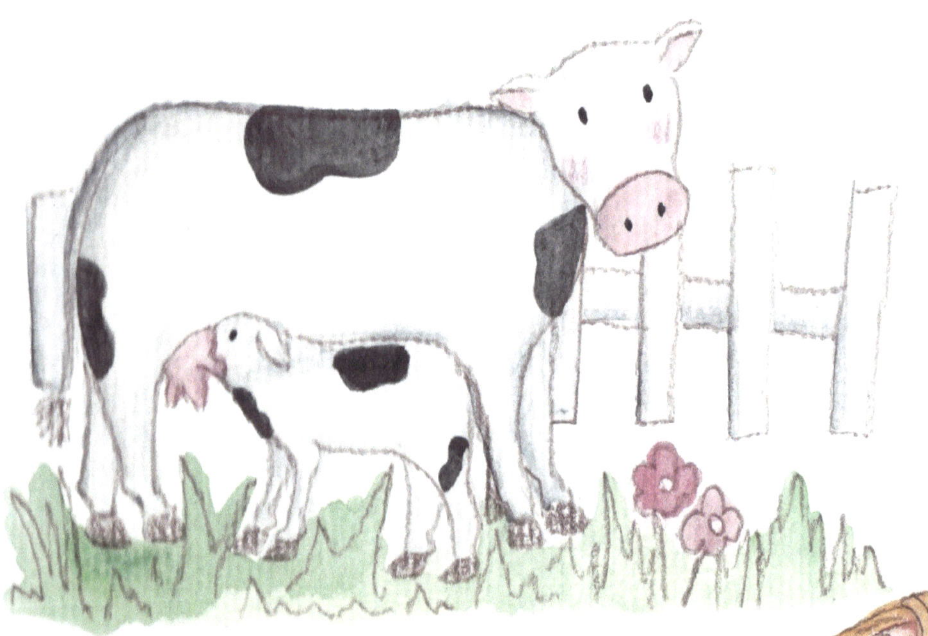

Stan leaves the milk
for the little baby cow
to drink.

He enjoys a glass of
refreshing water right
from the sink.

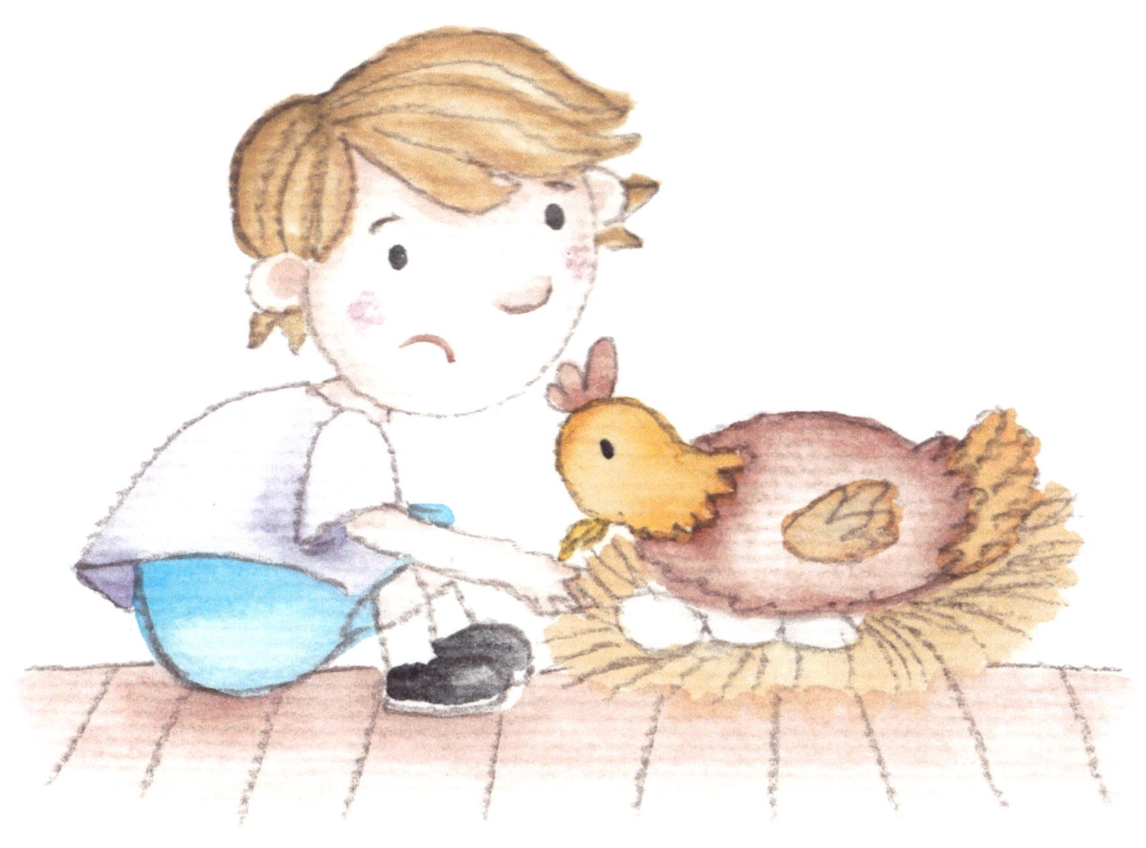

Stan knows hurting animals would not be kind to do.

This includes stealing from them too.

Stan sees all the colorful and furry animals as his friends.

He loves them all: cows, turkeys, pigs, and hens.

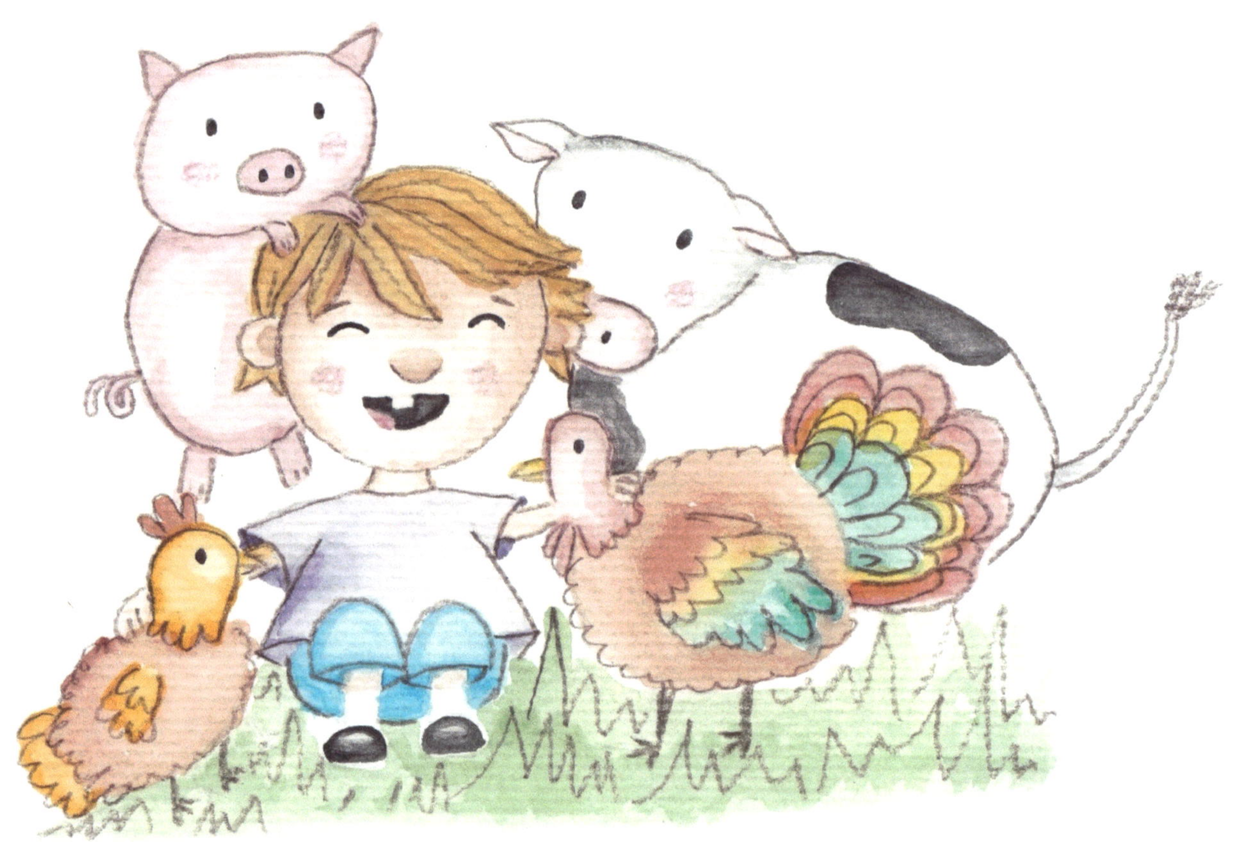

Stan could laugh and play with them all day long.

He will run, jump, roll around and sing a song.

Stan finds loving animals and eating plants to be so much fun.

He shares this beautiful message with everyone.

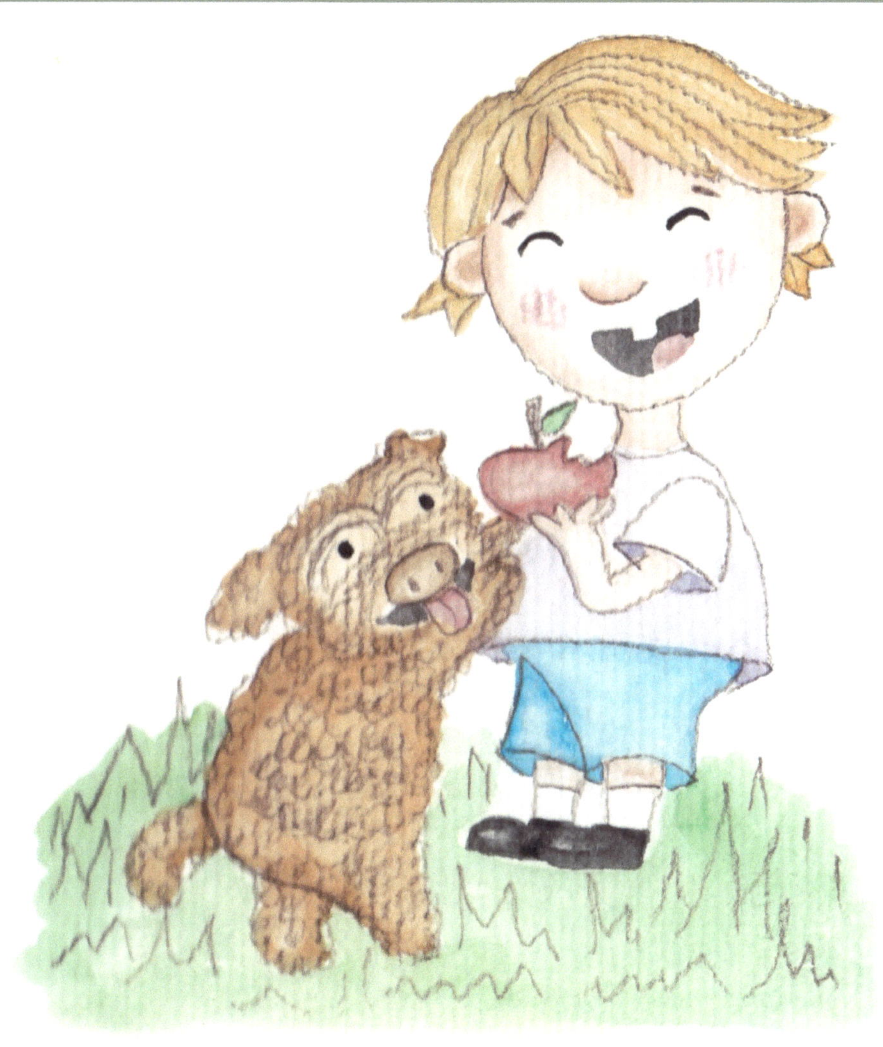

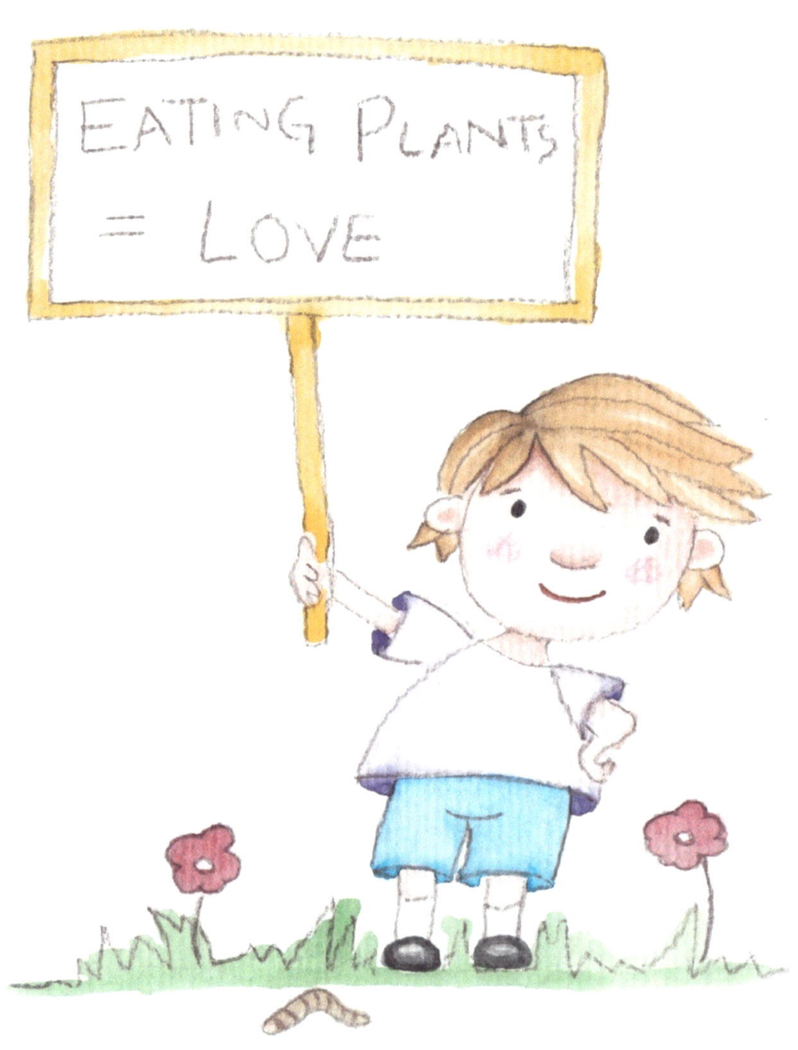
EATING PLANTS
= LOVE

About the Author

Stephen Bedwell Jr. is a Certified Holistic Nutrition Practitioner who educates children to eat a healthy whole food plant-based diet and encourages children to be environmentally friendly. He achieves this through creative and poetic stories that tug at the hearts and minds of children. Stephen lives in Wisconsin where he enjoys planting fruit trees and growing different types of herbs in his giant spiral in the woods.

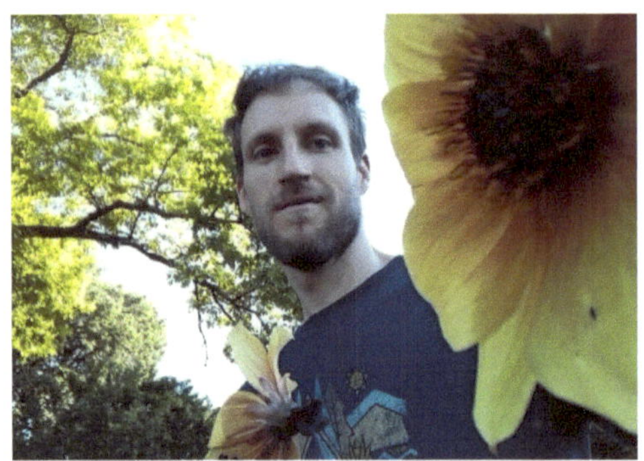